Table Of Contents

CW00509784

Introduction
The Circadian Cycle
The Sleep Cycle   14
How much is enough sleep?   18
Common Issues   20
Stress and Sleep   24
Creating the Right Environment   30
Creating a Bedtime Routine   38
Aromatherapy for Sleep   48
Sleep Quiz   56
Daily Planner   60
Weekly Success   67
Monthly Tracker   68
Affirmation Cards   69
Journal   70
Essential Oil Safety   72
Essential Oil Usage   78
Thank You!   80

The advice presented here is for information/ educational purposes and not a substitute for medical advice.

A health professional should always be consulted if symptoms persist or are serious.

External links/recommendations may be affiliate links whereby I earn a small percentage on any purchases you make through that website at no extra cost to you.

Hi and Welcome!

I'm a Massage and Complementary Therapist with over fifteen years experience. I've traveled the world to train with some of the most respected therapy teachers and schools. I've worked in a variety of settings including high-end spas, festivals and mental health charities. My passion is improving the quality of life for my clients; whether that be reducing stress, enhancing performance or managing a long-term health condition. I'm a firm believer in self-care; when we make clear improvements in our lives, it not only benefits us, but also all of the other people who depend on us. In today's hectic lifestyles this should no longer be seen as selfish, but necessary. Over the years I've witnessed clients coming to me with common issues. This has inspired me to put my training and experience together and create these guides covering the issues I see regularly in my treatment room. It is my hope that by continuing with regular treatments and following some of the advice in these guides, that you will see real, positive changes occur in your health and well-being.

Let's start!

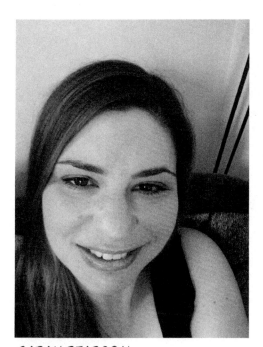

SARAH PEARSON

WELLNESS FACILITATOR

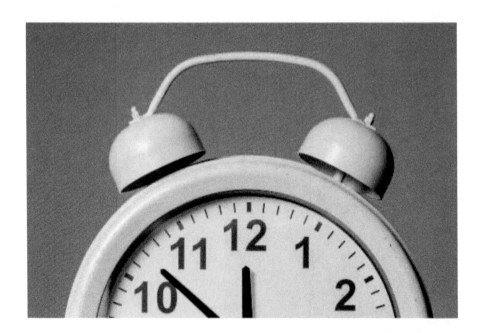

Introduction

Us humans spend around a third of our lives sleeping, yet scientists still don't fully understand why sleep is so essential to life. Numerous studies have shown the benefits of sleep and these include:

- Increased energy levels

- Increased mental clarity

- Improved memory and brain function

- Reduced stress and illness

- Helps the body's cells to repair

- Weight control

- Slows down the ageing process

- Improved skin and eye condition

According to the NHS website, it is estimated up to a third of adults will experience insomnia at some point. Studies have shown that the long-term effects of insomnia include an increased risk of:

- Diabetes

- Heart Attack

- High Blood Pressure

- Stroke

- Obesity

- Depression and Anxiety

As we can see, sleep has a huge impact on many of our bodies systems and our long-term health. Since a lot of the illnesses mentioned above are largely preventable, it can be argued that not getting enough sleep is a largely ignored Public Health issue. It follows therefore that improving our sleep is one of the easiest and important changes we can make to improving our health. Not only would this have repercussions on our quality of life but also for the NHS.

In this guide we will explore issues which can affect our sleep and simple measures we can take to improve it. Towards the back you will also find a worksheet section where you can be honest about your sleep issues, make a plan to resolve them and track your progress. It's easy to feel overwhelmed with all the health guidance we see online, the truth is we are all individuals and what works for one person won't necessarily work for someone else. Not all of the advice presented in this guide may be relevant to you, and changing too much at once means we are less likely to stick to new habits. Instead, I recommend making one or two changes at a time, continue if you feel they are working or drop them for a new habit if you feel they haven't made a difference. Use the tracking section to discover what really works for you and hopefully set you on a path to better sleep and a healthier you.

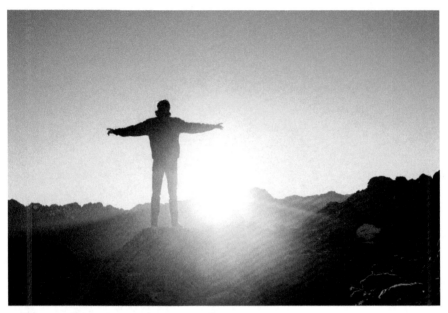

The Circadian Cycle

It's not my intention to get too weighed down with the science for the purpose of this guide. However I do believe two factors are important to understand in their role of sleep; the circadian cycle (or body clock) and the sleep cycle itself. By understanding these factors it is easier to pinpoint where issues may arise.

Put simply the Circadian Cycle is our body's natural internal body clock. Running on a 24-hour cycle, it tells us when to feel tired and when to feel alert. One of the ways it does this is by producing an organic compound called Adenosine. Our levels of Adenosine are at their lowest when we wake and increase for every hour we stay awake. Scientists believe this increase causes us to feel sleepy and less alert, thus telling us when to sleep. Adenosine is then broken down when we sleep for the cycle to continue.

Light also plays an important factor in the Circadian Cycle. Areas in the brain can differentiate between natural and artificial light, thus signalling day or night. As natural light fades, the hormone melatonin is released which makes us feel sleepy. When the sun rises in the morning, cortisol is released which makes us feel alert.

The Circadian cycle is the main reason why shift workers struggle with their sleep. Altering sleep patterns, needing to stay awake when it is dark and sleep during daylight make it difficult to settle into a routine and fight against the natural Circadian cycle. It is also the reason for jet lag when flying across time zones and why we feel 'out of sync' when the clocks change twice a year.

Other factors which may influence the Circadian Cycle or rhythm include medical conditions, medications, stress, sleep environment and certain foods and drinks. We are going to look into these in more detail later and see how we can influence our sleep with some simple changes.

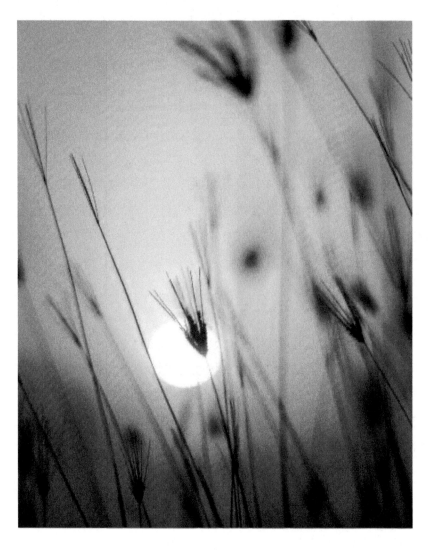

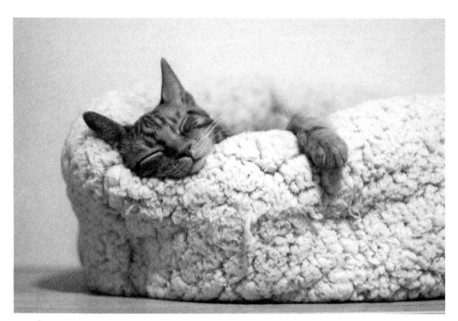

The Sleep Cycle

There are two main stages of sleep - Non Rapid Eye Movement (nREM) and Rapid Eye Movement (REM). Non Rapid Eye Movement is further broken down into three sections; stage one, two and three. These stages repeat cyclically throughout the night with stages of nREM becoming shorter and REM becoming longer.

Stage one nREM- The transition between being awake and asleep and usually consists of a couple of minutes of light sleep. I'm sure we've all had the feeling of waking and not knowing if we've been asleep or not - this is stage one. Muscles begin to relax, heart rate, breathing and eye movements slow down and our brain waves start to become less active.

Stage two nREM- The longest of the four sleep stages yet still classed as light sleep. Heart rate and breathing continue to slow down and body temperature begins to drop.

Stage three nREM - Deep sleep; heart rate, breathing and brain wave activity all fall to their lowest levels and it is difficult to wake up. During this stage the body repairs tissues, works on growth and development, boosts the immune system and builds energy. This stage is important to make us feel alert and refreshed the next day. This stage is longer at first and decreases in duration throughout the night.

Stage four REM - Made famous by the band, REM as the name suggests occurs when the eyes begin to move rapidly back and forth behind the eyes. Heart rate, breathing and blood pressure all increase and it is during this stage when we dream. The arms and legs also become paralysed and this is thought to be so that we don't act out on our dreams.

REM is also associated with turning our experiences into long-term memories. The length of REM increases throughout the night but also decreases as we get older. It is hard to wake during REM sleep and if we do we can feel unrefreshed and tired. Waking during this stage can also result in sleep paralysis as the limbs are still frozen. This can be quite frightening and disorienting for some people and therefore prevent them from fully experiencing REM sleep. However, it is important to remember that it is a perfectly normal situation and within seconds (although at the time may feel longer) the feeling will return.

By achieving the correct balance of each sleep cycle, we can be sure we are getting quality sleep. If you frequently wake feeling unrefreshed despite having achieved a full nights sleep then it is likely you're not spending enough time in stage three nREM for example. Knowing this means you can experiment with ways to improve this sleep stage.

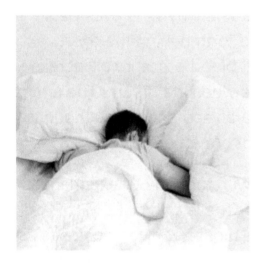

How much is enough sleep?

Recent research has shown that for most people middle-aged and older, seven hours seems to be the optimum amount of sleep. Younger people usually need more sleep. Traditionally it was believed that eight hours was the recommended amount and so personally I believe we should still aim for this. By doing so, if we have a 'bad night' or it takes longer to fall asleep, there is less pressure on getting the holy grail of seven hours.

I however am also a firm believer in everyone having different needs and finding what works for you. If you regularly have less sleep and function fine then that may be the right amount for you. If you're achieving eight hours but feel you need more, then perhaps you do need more than average. Please remember that 'average' is what we are talking about here so do not pressure yourself if you do not fit into that mould.

Discovering your optimum sleep amount is a prime example of learning to listen to your body (a mantra I often say to my clients!). The worksheets at the back of this guide will help you. However, we also need to recognise the difference between feeling tired because we need more sleep and feeling tired due to not being as alert. The latter can be caused by being bored, sitting for too long and dehydration. So before you start to think your afternoon slump is due to not having enough sleep; perhaps try taking a break from your desk, taking a walk, or having a glass of water.

I'm sure we've all experienced the occasional night where nothing we do makes us fall asleep, we lie awake for hours in a cycle of increasing frustration at not being able to sleep, which of course only makes it even more difficult to nod off. It is perfectly normal to have nights like this, however if it is happening regularly i.e. three nights a week or more, then it may be that you need to address the issue.

If you have been experiencing insomnia for more than a month and it is affecting your everyday life then it is time to see your GP. A common fear I hear is that the GP will prescribe them tablets which they do not wish to take, either because they only mask the problem or addiction worries. Sleeping pills are rarely prescribed these days and if so only for a short period of time as a last resort so please do not worry. You will more than likely be referred to a specialist sleep centre for assessment and help. Going to your appointment armed with the sleep diary at the back of this guide will give your clinicians a clear idea of what is going on and what you have tried.

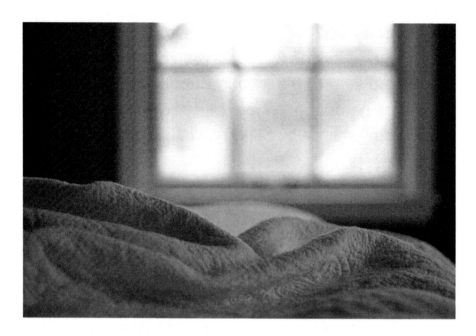

Common Issues

There are two main areas when it comes to sleep issues. The first is difficulty in falling asleep. The second is waking frequently, perhaps followed by struggling to get back to sleep. The former is often a result of poor bedtime habits, stress or simply not being tired enough to sleep. All of these factors we are going to address in this guide.

The latter is usually due to not falling into deep sleep or being easily disturbed. Again by following some of the principles on improving bedtime habits, you will hopefully fall deeper and stay asleep for longer. Unfortunately, as in life, some things keeping us awake are out of our control e.g. children, noisy housemates etc. Being as open and honest with members of your household about how lack of sleep is affecting you and what you need from them to help, maybe all it takes to improve their behaviour. However for things outside of your control, you may find some of the stress management tools relevant.

Numerous studies show that insomnia seems to affect women more than men. Whilst the reasons are unclear and could be social factors, for example young children being more likely to wake their Mum during the night, studies also show the quality of sleep can be affected by our monthly cycles.

During the latter half of our cycles, an increase in hormone activity can have a knock-on effect on our sleep. Have you ever woken in the night hot and sweaty around your time of the month? That's totally normal as body temperature often raises resulting in difficulty sleeping. Other issues can include stomach cramps and anxiety over leaks, both of which can result in keeping us awake.

Whilst not much extra can be done to specifically improve sleep around that time, keeping track of your cycle so that you're aware of any issues can help. By knowing your cycle you can pre-empt any issues and act accordingly; be stricter with your bedtime routine, wear cooler pyjamas and schedule your monthly reflexology treatment (or similar) for during that week are just some examples.

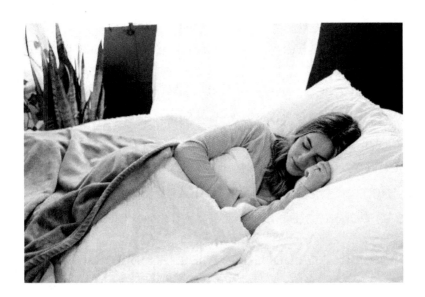

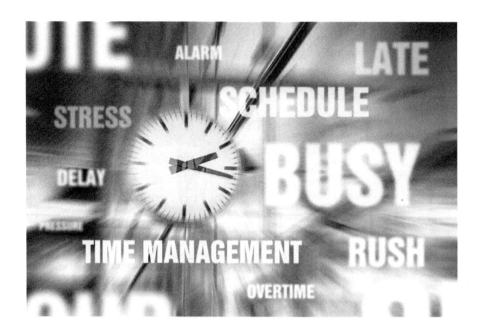

Stress and Sleep

We all experience stress from time to time, it's unavoidable. In fact a little bit of stress is actually good for us as the adrenaline it produces keeps us alert and motivated. Some people even strive on stress.

However prolonged exposure can have huge negative effects on the body with some scientists claiming stress is the contributing factor in 80% of all illnesses. It's easy to see why reducing our stress levels or at least learning some methods to improve our handling of stressful situations, can only have a positive effect on our health and wellbeing.

Poor sleep is a symptom of too much stress i.e. it is a sign for us to look out for and it is the stress which needs to be dealt with in order to improve our sleep. We can try all the lavender pillow sprays and herbal remedies known but without treating the underlying cause, little improvement will be made. Stress disrupts our sleep either because the act of worrying or overthinking is keeping us awake or the adrenaline itself is physically stopping us from falling asleep.

Stress management is a whole guide in itself, however these are my main ways to reduce stress when it is specifically impacting your sleep.

#1 WRITE IT DOWN

The same theory behind talking to a friend, only without the fear of judgement. Getting our fears, thoughts and emotions out on paper can have a releasing effect. It doesn't need to be a fancy journal, any random notepad will do or there is a worksheet at the back if you prefer. No one is going to read it so don't worry about spelling, grammar etc, it is your opportunity to fully express yourself, release your deepest fears and emotions you wouldn't dare to tell anyone. For some, seeing what they have written gives them an epiphany moment and they realise what has been bothering them is actually rather insignificant. For others, it is a starting point to create an action plan on how to resolve the issue. It doesn't matter what you do with it after, some people like to keep it and reflect later, others like to destroy it in a symbolic gesture of letting go. It is the act of getting these thoughts out of your head that is important.

#2 BREATHING EXERCISES

There are lots of different breathing exercises online. It really is personal preference which ones work for you so have a look on YouTube, try a couple and see what resonates with you. They all tend to have the same purpose; slowing down the mind and body, and focusing only on your breathing. Guided meditations have the same effect if you prefer those instead

#3 AFFIRMATIONS

Countless studies have shown that a positive mindset gives positive results. It is easier to see this by imagining the opposite. How many times have you been running late only to be held up even more by catching every red light on your route? Have you ever felt all the 'bad stuff' in your life seemed to happen in a short period of time? In reality when we dwell on something negative, it fuels recognition for further negativity and so the cycle continues. Lying in bed at night, fretting over not being able to sleep only fuels the idea that we cannot sleep.

Shifting our mindset into a positive one is not easy, it takes practice and this is where affirmations can help. Remembering and repeating a positive quote or saying, embeds it into our brains. Over the page are a few examples, pick one which resonates with you. You may wish to write it out and keep it by your bedside, make it into a meme as a screensaver on your phone or repeat it like a mantra as you try to fall asleep.

A blank version of these affirmation cards is available in the worksheet section to create your own.

EVERY DAY I AM GETTING HEALTHIER.

SLEEP COMES EASY TO ME.

I ACCEPT SLEEP INTO MY LIFE.

I AM DESERVING OF A PEACEFUL NIGHTS SLEEP.

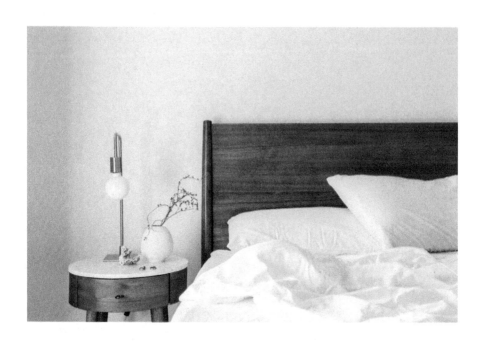

Creating the Right Environment

When we are younger most of us take sleep for granted, as such bad habits creep in. Most of the time we don't even realise these habits could be the cause of our poor sleep. Creating a sleep environment is often neglected, however on a subconscious level it sends important signals to the brain, allowing it to switch off much easier. The more we repeat these behaviours, the more our brain associates them with sleep.

If you have ever had a treatment with me, you will know I often use the same music and the same aromas because it underpins the same theory;

repeated habits allow the brain to recognise it is time to switch off; it is a time for nurturing and comfort, a safe space. Getting into bed should conjure up these same emotions for you.

One of the main issues people do not realise can have a detrimental effect on their sleep is their sleep environment. The bedroom should be a place of calm and tranquility, a sanctuary where we feel most at peace. If the last thing you see before turning off the light are piles of clutter, dirty laundry or stacks of paperwork, then the brain is thinking of all the things you need to do rather than being conducive to sleep.

Take a good look around your bedroom and be honest with yourself; what doesn't need to be there? What can be moved to another room, stored better or thrown away? Be ruthless and streamline the contents of the room to the bare minimum you need.

This moves me to my next point; the bedroom should be for sleeping only! (And other nocturnal activities but more on that later!) This means moving the tv from the room, no eating and no working from bed on the laptop. All of these activities are too stimulating for the bedroom and do not create the right sleep environment. If this isn't possible for example because you live in a studio apartment or lodging in a shared house, then try to create a barrier, ideally a curtain, screen or room divider of some kind, to partition the sleep area from the activity area.

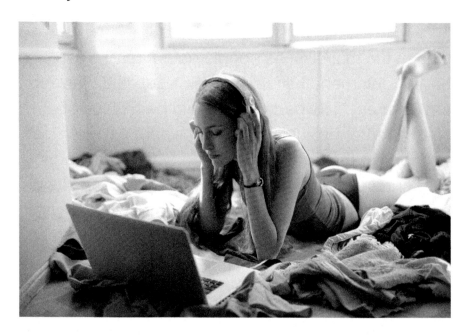

Moving on to your bed itself; Have your mattress and/or pillows seen better days? Are they still comfy and are they giving you the right support? Choosing the right mattress and pillows is a bit of a lottery, I wish there was a 'one size fits all' approach to them. Finding the right items for you depends on a number of factors including whether you sleep on your side, front or back,; the shape of your spine; the breadth of your shoulders. Many mattress retailers now have technology whereby they can test your pressure points and find the best one for you. Mattresses are expensive but since we spend a third of our lives laying on one they are worth the investment. It is worth seeking an expert opinion and utilising free trials to make sure it is right for you.

Pillows are a little more complicated as there is no technology (that I know of) which will give you recommendations and on such relatively low value items we are not likely to get any soon. Just because a pillow is expensive or memory foam does not mean it will be suitable for you. The key with pillows is to make sure your head and neck are in alignment. Too much or too little support will lead to the neck bending and over time cause tension in the neck muscles, this often then extends into shoulders or causes tension headaches. For me as a massage therapist, incorrect pillows for your head/shoulder shape is the number one reason clients come to me with neck issues. If you are waking up with pain in the neck which eases as the day progresses, it is a telltale sign that your pillows need addressing. Which one you choose and how many you use really is a case of trial and error - sorry!

Next on the list of creating the right environment is avoiding screens in the bedroom. I've already mentioned removing the tv from the room but this extends to mobile phones, tablets, and laptops. We all know that using screens before bed stimulates the brain and makes it harder to fall asleep, but even when the screens are 'off' the appliances themselves emit a type of light that can also be stimulating. Plus removing them from the room means the temptation to use them is also gone. Again they are not conducive to sleep so have no place in the bedroom! If you must keep your phone with you during the night, switch it to 'do not disturb' mode. This is better than just 'silent' as the screen won't light up with every message or notification. Check your settings as most still allow you to select phone calls from certain numbers to come through so you won't miss any emergency calls.

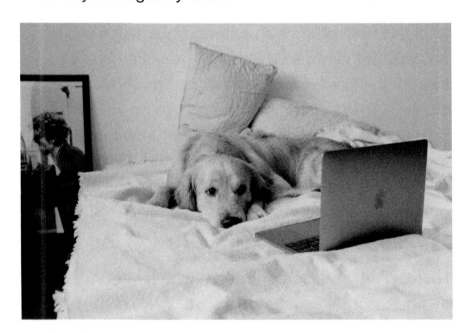

Avoiding noise is also an often cited recommendation. However for some this is unavoidable, living near a busy road or a snoring partner for example. If you feel that noise is disturbing you and can't be stopped then you may wish to consider ear plugs. For some people however noise can be soothing, white noise for example or gentle music. This can block out any distracting noise but for some may also be a positive behaviour which induces sleep. Experiment and see which works for you.

Any light, tricks the brain into thinking it is daytime and so can affect sleep. Use blackout blinds or curtains and avoid nightlights. If light is inevitable e.g. a street light right outside your bedroom window, or working nights means you are sleeping during daylight hours or even noticing you are waking earlier in summer when the sun rises earlier, then you may wish to consider using an eye mask.

Recent research has actually shown that even if we are unaware light is keeping us awake, wearing an eye mask could still be beneficial to our sleep.(1)

1. Source: Viviano Greco et al. Sept 2023 Wearing an Eye Mask During Overnight Sleep Improves Episodic Learning and Alertness. PubMed

Participants in a recent study reported they were more alert and showed improved learning following wearing an eye-mask to sleep. It is believed being in complete darkness increased their deep sleep, thus improving their quality of sleep. So if you frequently wake feeling unrefreshed, try using an eye-mask for a week and see if you notice a difference

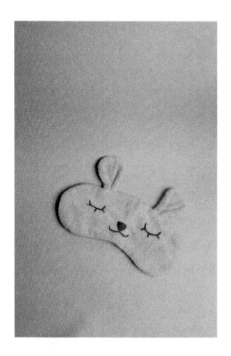

Whilst on the subject of light, if you struggle to wake in the morning, then you may wish to invest in a light 'alarm' clock. As we discovered earlier, waking unrefreshed is often the result of waking during the

deep sleep cycle. These light boxes mimic the rising sun by gradually getting brighter the closer to the time you set. This tricks the brain into waking you naturally by bringing you out of deep sleep first before waking fully. There are several on the market, some even combine aromatherapy diffusers and radio so do your own research for one which matches your needs and budget. Of course they're probably not conducive if you wear a sleep mask and so it's another example of deciding which is right for you and your circumstances!

There have been numerous studies and research which indicate the colour of a bedroom can affect a person's sleep. Muted, darker shades of blues and greens seem to promote the best sleepers. Respondents claimed colours which reminded them of nature invoked calmness and serenity, thus helping them to sleep. Whereas colours to avoid are purple, brown and grey. Personally, I think there are larger factors which are easier to change if you are committed to improving your sleep. I'm not going to advocate redecorating and I appreciate for renters there may not be a choice in your decor, but if you are planning on decorating your bedroom it may be something to consider. (Source: Does room colour affect serenity and quality of sleep? Han Gao University of Richmond)

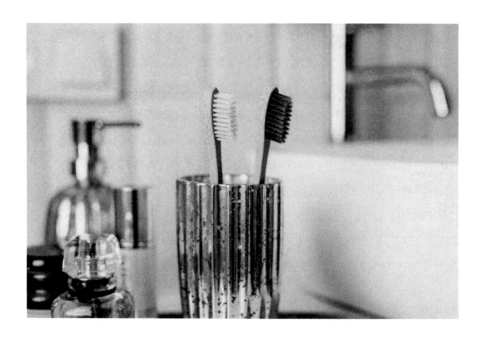

Creating a Bedtime Routine

If you have young kids or if not remember when you were young; you will understand the importance of a regular bedtime routine. We cut out sugary drinks and snacks and do nothing too stimulating; a bath and bedtime story is as exciting as post-7 pm life gets for a six-year-old.

The freedom of being an adult is that we do as we please without consequence; stay up late playing computer games or watching one more episode of a Netflix box-set; drinking and eating to excess or simply catching up with people or errands from the day. Any bedtime routine is long-forgotten and we go to bed hyped and then try to unwind. It's no wonder that going to bed in that hyped-up state means it takes longer to get to sleep, and as we've seen before the anxiety struggling to get to sleep creates, only fuels the cycle of insomnia further.

As we discussed in the previous chapter, I'm a fan of routine; repeated positive behaviours and habits send signals to the brain so it recognises what to do i.e. in this case, sleep. It should come as no surprise therefore that I strongly advise putting a regular bedtime routine in place. For one hour before bed, only do activities which are going to help you unwind and therefore promote sleep, and repeat this every night. The following is an example of a bedtime routine, but experiment, see what works for you and feel free to add your own suggestions-

1. Switch off all screens (no tv, phones, iPads or laptops)

2. Have a bath

3. Conduct your nightly skin care routine

4. Spend ten minutes doing some yoga/pilates/ stretches

5. Meditate

6. Write your journal/tomorrows 'to do' list

7. Read (nothing you're too engrossed in or a crime thriller; the less you need to focus the better!)

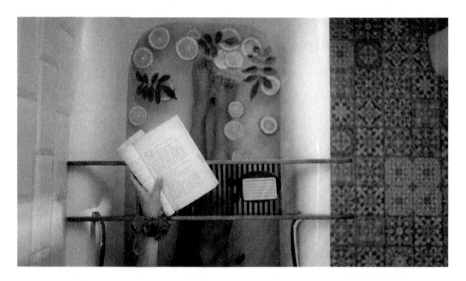

Personally, I keep a tube of hand cream by my bed so that the last thing I do before turning out the light is apply some and give myself a short hand massage. My hands are literally the tools of my trade and are constantly being washed which means it's pointless applying any during the day. This small ritual for me, signifies my day is over and rewards my hands for their hard-work. What small ritual can you include in your nighttime routine? Something small but significant to you and your lifestyle.

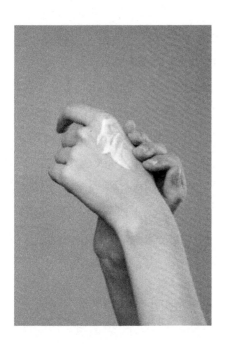

There are a plethora of supplements on the market claiming to improve sleep. Personally, I'm not a fan of supplements and it is beyond my scope to recommend any. Unless you have certain medical conditions, if you are eating a well-balanced diet and avoiding the usual items on the naughty list (be honest we all know what we should and shouldn't be eating!) then there is usually no need to be taking supplements. If you do decide to go down that path, please speak to a qualified herbalist who will check for interactions with any other medications you may be taking and find the right remedy personalised for you. Evidence on any supplements' effectiveness however is limited and they are usually not recommended to be used long-term, hence another reason why I do not advise using them. A bit like sleeping pills, they should only be used when necessary and not relied on. If you really want to experiment with the herbal route, try herbal teas as a starting point. Several brands offer a sleep blend (my personal favourite is Aldi!) Some key ingredients to look out for are Chamomile, Passionflower and Valerian. These have the added benefit of being both sugar and caffeine-free so are perfect if you like a hot drink before bed.

One element it may be worth considering to improve sleep is Magnesium. Magnesium deficiency is difficult to diagnose and therefore is likely to be under reported though is believed to be common in the UK. Signs of a deficiency can be muscle cramps and restless legs, symptoms often reported as keeping people awake at night. It also has a calming effect and so studies have shown that if stress or anxiety are keeping you awake, then Magnesium may help improve sleep. One of the best ways to increase Magnesium in the body is actually through skin absorption. Epsom salts (i.e. Magnesium Sulphate to give them their scientific name!) added to the bath is a great way to top-up your Magnesium levels. Alternatively there are body creams and sprays containing Magnesium, some of my clients have had particularly good results with the oil spray for muscle aches, cramps and restless legs sprayed directly onto the affected areas.

Now it's time to discuss our bedtime and wake time. Unless you're retired, your wake time will probably be dictated to by work, school or child commitments. Ideally we should work backwards and subtract eight hours from our wake time to determine our ideal bedtime. However as we know, everyone is different, so if you're lying awake staring at the ceiling for hours and you're simply not tired then going to bed that early is pointless, it will only fuel sleep anxiety. It sounds simple but if you're not tired then don't go to bed! Similarly if you're falling asleep on the sofa before your 'bedtime' then it's likely you need to go to bed earlier. A common complaint is falling asleep on the sofa and then being wide awake when getting to bed. A possible reason for this, is the action of going upstairs, getting ready for bed etc has woken you up and now your mind is no longer in 'sleep mode'. An earlier bedtime will pre-empt this and make sure when you fall asleep you are able to stay asleep.

It is important to try and keep to the same bedtime and wake time as much as possible. We're all guilty of having late-nights or lie-ins on a weekend, but deviating from our usual times by more than an hour disrupts the body clock and makes it harder when we need to revert back to our usual routine. The same principles lie around napping during the day. It is generally not advised as again disrupts our circadian rhythm the same way as sleeping on the sofa. If you find yourself napping frequently, it should be seen as a sign you are not sleeping enough at night and perhaps need to try an earlier bedtime.

Many people fall into the trap of thinking they can 'catch up' on lost sleep during the weekend. Not only does this have the effect of disrupting the Circadian rhythm as above, but we don't really have a sleep 'deficit' to catch up on. Experts are in agreement that the logic of 'catching up' on sleep doesn't work and our focus should be getting an equal amount of sleep each night.

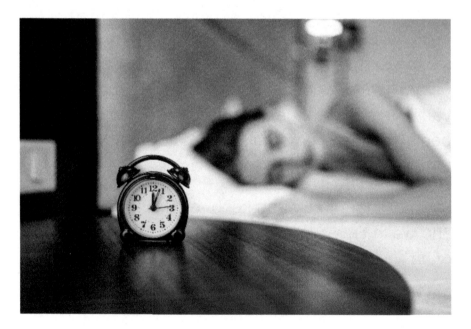

Since we have discussed things we should do before bed, it is now time to discuss things to avoid. Firstly is stimulants, these prevent the formation of adenosine (remember the sleepy chemical we discussed in the introduction?) thus keeping us too alert and so should be avoided. Examples include nicotine (in any form, cigarettes vapes etc) and recreational drugs. Some medication can also disrupt sleep but please discuss this with your GP if you feel this is the case. They may be able to switch you to an alternative, do not stop taking any prescribed medication without consulting with them first.

Caffeine also prevents adenosine production and so should also be limited before bed. However, everyone has different tolerances to caffeine and so it is best to work out your own cut-off time. I've seen some experts recommend no caffeine after 5pm, whilst others as early as midday. If you think caffeine is impacting your sleep, experiment by choosing a cut- off time and stick to it for a week. If you see no improvement bring your cut-off time forward by an hour and repeat until you find your optimum time.

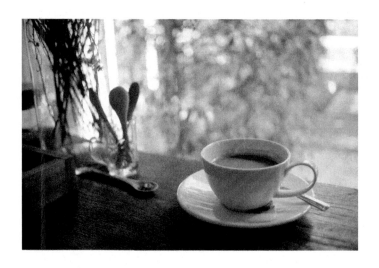

Many people like to have an alcoholic drink before bed as they say it relaxes them and so helps them get to sleep. Whilst that may be true, once alcohol is broken down it actually becomes a stimulant and so whilst it may help you get to sleep, often you will then wake or become restless during the night. I would therefore recommend avoiding alcohol in the hours leading up to bedtime. Drinking earlier in the day means that by the time you head to bed, alcohol has entered its' stimulant phase. I hate to sound like a party pooper but limiting alcohol and not drinking to excess can have a profound benefit on our health.

Another activity that is often too stimulating right before bed is exercise. Whilst stretching is recommended, cardio or weights i.e. any activity which is going to raise the heart rate is best to avoid. Keep any strenuous activity to earlier in the day to use up surplus energy and burn calories. In fact exercise during the day can actually improve sleep by tiring out the body. The only exception to this exercise rule you will be pleased to hear is sex. Yes, there is a reason sex is usually reserved as a nocturnal activity, having an orgasm releases all kinds of relaxing, happy hormones helping to send us off to sleep. So whether it be on your own or with a partner, I'm sure that's one pre-bedtime ritual we can all stick to!

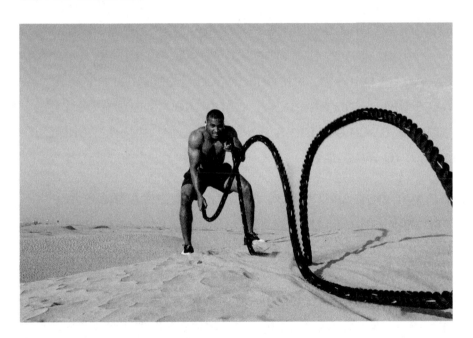

Aromatherapy for Sleep

When using Essential oils for sleep you can try diffusing them in your bedroom, add them to your bath or use a pillow spray. Essential oils are complex chemical compounds which are believed to have a physical effect on the body. Some have a relaxing effect, others balance hormones, aid digestion or energise for example. Scent however is also closely linked to memory, I'm sure we've all experienced instances of a perfume taking us back to a memory of a night out or the smell of certain cooking aromas taking us back to our childhood. Essential oils can have the same effect, by using them before bed the brain associates the smell as time to sleep making it easier to switch off.

It's also however a good idea to change the oils you use regularly so that you don't become sensitive to the oil. So try having two or three of your favourites on rotation. Essential oils are more than just great smells and should be used with caution and only when needed. For more guidance on the correct usage of oils, please see the Essential Oil appendix.

When mentioning essential oils which help sleep, one oil always comes to mind; Lavender. It's such a cliche and so many clients tell me they hate it that

I've devised a list of my top five essential oils to help promote sleep which does not include Lavender! Of course, if it's your favourite and works for you then carry on using it, but if you do want to try some alternatives then these are the ones I suggest.

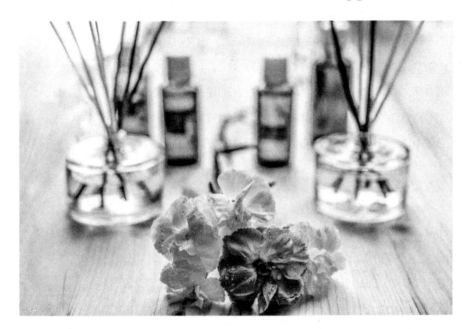

Top Five Essential Oils for Sleep

Petitgrain

One of my favourite essential oils, and I would argue the best (including Lavender!) when it comes to promoting sleep. It comes from the leaves of the bitter orange tree and therefore has a herbal scent but with a subtle orange after-note. Particularly calming and comforting in times of loneliness.

Valerian

More commonly used as a herbal tincture or in teas as a sedative to promote sleep. I've included the essential oil here as an alternative to taking remedies, although the essential oil is more expensive compared to the others listed here. It is however a useful oil for restlessness and has a pleasant musky aroma which many prefer.

Sweet Marjoram

Calming on the nervous system this is another oil beneficial for stress and anxiety. However it is highly potent and can be an anaphrodisiac so caution is recommended - definitely an oil to be used when needed rather than daily!

Roman Chamomile

One of the gentlest essential oils, it is particularly soothing and recommended for insomnia where stress and anxiety are the underlying causes. It has a distinctive 'earthy' smell and so is best blended with a floral or citrus oil to lift the scent.

Lemon Balm/Melissa

The smell of Melissa essential oil reminds me of lemon sherbet! Like Lemon (which you could also use if you struggle to find Melissa, though I find lemon quite stimulating, Melissa is much more subtle and therefore better for sleep) it calms an over-active mind. But it is particularly beneficial during times of trauma or grief. So if over-thinking is making you toss and turn, or you're going through a tough time, then Melissa may be an oil to turn to. Just be careful applying it to your skin as it can irritate some people.

Make your own Pillow Mist

Aromatherapy pillow sprays have gained in popularity in recent years, however a quick glance at the ingredient list and most are barely more than Lavender water. So here I'm going to share my recipe to make your own for a fraction of the price and you can vary the oils to suit your taste. Experiment with different oils/water combinations and make some extra, they make perfect handmade gifts for friends and family.

You will need-

-100 ml spray bottle

-Approx 95ml of oral water*/ distilled water (boiled and cooled is acceptable for home use) - use a combination to dilute the oral water if you prefer

- 2-3mls of essential oils (unless you have a talent for blending smells, stick to one/two at most)

-1ml Vitamin E (this extends the shelf life, if you don't want the expense of buying a bottle, get some capsules from a health food shop, pierce and squeeze in the liquid from one capsule)

-2-3mls of Polysorbate 80 (this allows the water and oil to mix, available from diy skincare retailers such as 'Naturally Thinking' you can exclude it but you will need to shake your spray vigorously each time before you use) You could also use a teaspoon of Vodka if that's easier to get hold of!

*A by-product from the distillation process to make essential oils, sometimes referred to as a hydrosol or hydrolat, available from aromatherapy retailers. Lavender is commonly used for a pillow spray but you could also try neroli/orange flower or rose water as a cheaper alternative to using their essential oils.

Method
Add all ingredients to your bottle, shake and viola! It's as easy as that! Spritz 2-3 sprays over your pillows each night. Since it is the scent which is linked to our memory and is reminding us to sleep, remember to pack your spray if you are sleeping away for the night.

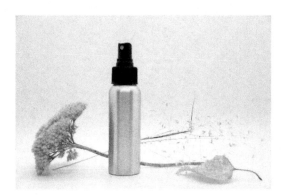

Over to You...

It's all well and good reading advice but without clear planning and reflection, we are less likely to put this advice into action. The following pages contain several planners and quizzes to analyse and track your sleep.

Of course, there are several gadgets and apps available which can track your sleep. By all means, use them if you prefer however for some they can fuel sleep anxiety in the same way constantly checking a clock can. So if you're less tech-savvy or are committed to keeping screens out of the bedroom then print off the following pages to fill in the good old- fashioned way!

For a printable version of these worksheets please use the QR code over the page

www.leru-wellness.co.uk

Sleep QUIZ

WHAT ARE YOUR MAIN SLEEP ISSUES?

Difficulty falling asleep.

Difficulty staying asleep

Partner/children/pets waking me up

Snoring/breathing issues

Other (please state)

DO YOU AWAKEN REFRESHED?

Always

Almost always

Sometimes

Rarely

Never

DO YOU KEEP A REGULAR SLEEP SCHEDULE?

Bed time?
....

Wake time?
....

ONCE IN BED HOW LONG DOES IT TAKE YOU TO SLEEP?

HOW MANY TIMES DO YOU WAKE EACH NIGHT?

Sleep QUIZ

HOW MUCH SLEEP DO YOU LOSE DUE TO FREQUENT WAKING?

WHAT CAUSES YOU TO WAKE?

Partner/children/pets /noise

Needing the toilet

Light sleeper

Other

HOW LONG DOES IT TAKE FOR YOU TO BE FULLY AWAKE?

HOW OFTEN DO YOU TAKE NAPS? (INCLUDE FALLING ASLEEP ACCIDENTLY OF AN EVENING!)

Daily

Rarely

Never

HOW LONG ARE YOUR NAPS?

WHEN FREE TO CHOOSE, WHAT TIME DO YOU PREFER TO GO TO SLEEP?

WHAT TIME WOULD YOU PREFER TO WAKE?

Sleep QUIZ

DO YOU CONSUME ANY OF THE FOLLOWING DAILY?

Caffeine

Alcohol

Tobacco

Mood altering drugs (prescribed and illegal)

DO ANY BLOOD RELATIVES ALSO HAVE SLEEP ISSUES?

daily PLANNER

Pre-bed Routine

_____

_____

_____

_____

Add the following to the
schedule on the right

Wake time

Nap time

Exercise (when and what?)

Last meal

Last caffeine

Last alcoholic
drink/cigarette/other as
applicable

Bed time

Sleep time

	6 AM
	7 AM
	8 AM
	9 AM
	10 AM
	11 AM
	12 PM
	1 PM
	2 PM
	3 PM
	4 PM
	5 PM
	6 PM
	7 PM
	8 PM
	9 PM
	10 PM
	11 PM
	12 AM
	1 AM
	2 AM
	3 AM
	4 AM

HOW DID I FEEL ON WAKING?

Refreshed

Still tired

TODAYS ENERGY

1 2 3 4 5

TODAYS MOOD:

1 2 3 4 5

RATE LAST NIGHTS SLEEP

1 2 3 4 5

Why have you given these scores?

daily PLANNER

DATE: TUESDAY

6 AM
7 AM
8 AM
9 AM
10 AM
11 AM
12 PM
1 PM
2 PM
3 PM
4 PM
5 PM
6 PM
7 PM
8 PM
9 PM
10 PM
11 PM
12 AM
1 AM
2 AM
3 AM
4 AM

Pre-bed Routine

_____

_____

_____

_____

Add the following to the schedule on the right

Wake time

Nap time

Exercise (when and what?)

Last meal

Last caffeine

Last alcoholic drink/cigarette/other as applicable

Bed time

Sleep time

HOW DID I FEEL ON WAKING?

Refreshed

Still tired

TODAYS ENERGY

1   2   3   4   5

TODAYS MOOD:

1   2   3   4   5

RATE LAST NIGHTS SLEEP

1   2   3   4   5

Why have you given these scores?

www.leru-wellness.co.uk

daily PLANNER

	6 AM
	7 AM
Pre-bed Routine	8 AM
_____	9 AM
	10 AM
_____	11 AM
	12 PM
_____	1 PM
	2 PM
_____	3 PM
Add the following to the schedule on the right	4 PM
Wake time	5 PM
Nap time	6 PM
Exercise (when and what?)	7 PM
Last meal	8 PM
Last caffeine	9 PM
Last alcoholic drink/cigarette/other as applicable	10 PM
	11 PM
Bed time	12 AM
Sleep time	1 AM
	2 AM
	3 AM
	4 AM

HOW DID I FEEL ON WAKING?

Refreshed

Still tired

TODAYS ENERGY

1 2 3 4 5

TODAYS MOOD:

1 2 3 4 5

RATE LAST NIGHTS SLEEP

1 2 3 4 5

Why have you given these scores?

daily PLANNER

	6 AM
	7 AM
Pre-bed Routine	8 AM
_____	9 AM
	10 AM
_____	11 AM
	12 PM
_____	1 PM
	2 PM
_____	
Add the following to the schedule on the right	3 PM
	4 PM
Wake time	5 PM
Nap time	6 PM
Exercise (when and what?)	7 PM
Last meal	8 PM
Last caffeine	9 PM
Last alcoholic drink/cigarette/other as applicable	10 PM
	11 PM
Bed time	12 AM
Sleep time	1 AM
	2 AM
	3 AM
	4 AM

HOW DID I FEEL ON WAKING?

Refreshed

Still tired

TODAYS ENERGY

1 2 3 4 5

TODAYS MOOD:

1 2 3 4 5

RATE LAST NIGHTS SLEEP

1 2 3 4 5

Why have you given these scores?

daily PLANNER

6 AM	
7 AM	
8 AM	
9 AM	
10 AM	
11 AM	
12 PM	
1 PM	
2 PM	
3 PM	
4 PM	
5 PM	
6 PM	
7 PM	
8 PM	
9 PM	
10 PM	
11 PM	
12 AM	
1 AM	
2 AM	
3 AM	
4 AM	

Pre-bed Routine

_____

_____

_____

_____

Add the following to the schedule on the right

Wake time

Nap time

Exercise (when and what?)

Last meal

Last caffeine

Last alcoholic drink/cigarette/other as applicable

Bed time

Sleep time

HOW DID I FEEL ON WAKING?

Refreshed

Still tired

TODAYS ENERGY

1 2 3 4 5

TODAYS MOOD:

1 2 3 4 5

RATE LAST NIGHTS SLEEP

1 2 3 4 5

Why have you given these scores?

daily PLANNER

Pre-bed Routine

_____

_____

_____

_____

Add the following to the
schedule on the right

Wake time

Nap time

Exercise (when and what?)

Last meal

Last caffeine

Last alcoholic
drink/cigarette/other as
applicable

Bed time

Sleep time

6 AM	
7 AM	
8 AM	
9 AM	
10 AM	
11 AM	
12 PM	
1 PM	
2 PM	
3 PM	
4 PM	
5 PM	
6 PM	
7 PM	
8 PM	
9 PM	
10 PM	
11 PM	
12 AM	
1 AM	
2 AM	
3 AM	
4 AM	

HOW DID I FEEL ON WAKING?

Refreshed

Still tired

TODAYS ENERGY

1 2 3 4 5

TODAYS MOOD:

1 2 3 4 5

RATE LAST NIGHTS SLEEP

1 2 3 4 5

Why have you given these scores?

daily PLANNER

6 AM	
7 AM	
8 AM	
9 AM	
10 AM	
11 AM	
12 PM	
1 PM	
2 PM	
3 PM	
4 PM	
5 PM	
6 PM	
7 PM	
8 PM	
9 PM	
10 PM	
11 PM	
12 AM	
1 AM	
2 AM	
3 AM	
4 AM	

Pre-bed Routine

_____

_____

_____

_____

Add the following to the
schedule on the right

Wake time

Nap time

Exercise (when and what?)

Last meal

Last caffeine

Last alcoholic
drink/cigarette/other as
applicable

Bed time

Sleep time

HOW DID I FEEL ON WAKING?

Refreshed

Still tired

TODAYS ENERGY

(1) (2) (3) (4) (5)

TODAYS MOOD:

(1) (2) (3) (4) (5)

RATE LAST NIGHTS SLEEP

(1) (2) (3) (4) (5)

Why have you given these
scores?

weekly SUCCESS

REVIEW YOUR WEEK, AND MAKE SURE TO COMPLETE THE
QUESTIONS BELOW IN FULL.

HOW MANY NIGHTS OF FULFILLING SLEEP HAVE I HAD?

WHAT CHANGES HAVE I MADE?

WHAT HAVE I LEARNED THIS WEEK?

WHAT AM I GRATEFUL FOR THIS WEEK?

WHAT ONE THING COULD I DO DIFFERENTLY NEXT WEEK?

monthly TRACKER

MONTH:

Sometimes it helps to see the bigger picture so use this tracker to view how many hours of sleep you have had each night over a month. Ladies, you may also wish to mark on the tracker the first day of your menstrual cycle to see if that impacts your sleep.

Sun	Mon	Tues	Wed	Thurs	Fri	Sat

affirmation CARDS

Print these affirmation cards and write your own affirmations. Remember to use positive language only and avoid the word 'not' e.g. 'I will not wake during the night' becomes 'I will sleep soundly throughout the night'

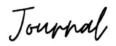

Journal

USE THIS SPACE TO WRITE YOUR WORRIES/FEARS/TO DO LIST
KEEPING YOU AWAKE

ITEM 1:   ITEM 2:   ITEM 3:

ACTIONS TO   ACTIONS TO   ACTIONS TO
OVERCOME: OVERCOME: OVERCOME:

_____   _____   _____

_____   _____   _____

_____   _____   _____

_____   _____   _____

_____   _____   _____

_____   _____   _____

Essential Oil Safety

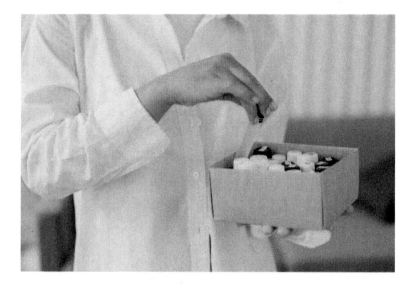

There has been a huge increase in the use of essential oils in recent years. This is partly due to well- meaning bloggers and social media claiming cheap and effective cures for any ailment. However with that, has come a myriad of sales lies, dangerous misinformation and even hospitalisations due to misuse. As a professional and qualified Aromatherapist, I feel it is my duty to include the following guidelines when advising people to use essential oils at home. If you are in any doubt however, please seek advice from a qualified aromatherapist, we undertake thorough training in the safety aspect of using essential oils and it is in our interest to raise the standard and respect of the aromatherapy industry. Retailers however, have received little to no training and are often only interested in making a sale!

Firstly when it comes to buying oils, always chose a respectable retailer. There are several online but my personal favourites are 'Naturally Thinking' or 'Base Formula'. Both sell good quality essential oils and associated products at a reasonable price. Beware of oils which seem cheap, they are often fragrance oils i.e. they smell the same as the oil but do not have the therapeutic qualities of an essential oil, or have already been diluted down. Oils should usually come in a dark, glass bottle and have a dropper. These are all to preserve the oil for as long as possible. Oils do have a shelf-life, although usually not considered harmful, they may not smell their best or lose some of their therapeutic value if past their best. If an oil is thicker, smells different or if crystals are forming around the thread of the bottle top, then consider replacing that oil. Oils should ideally be stored in a cool, dark place e.g. in a cupboard and never in direct sunlight as this speeds up the degradation process.

There is so much more to essential oils than just smelling good. They are extracted from plants and as such are concentrated, complex chemicals. Essential oils should never be used undiluted directly on the skin nor should they be taken internally i.e. added to a pill or worse diluted in water to drink. I often see or hear comments such as 'but if the oil is pure/organic then what is the harm?' The issue is not the purity of the oil, but the fact that as we have previously stated, essential oils are complex, concentrated, chemical compounds. Repeated exposure can cause sensitivities such as rashes and blisters. Plus oil and water do not mix, adding oil to water and then drinking it still means undiluted oil can come into contact with your stomach lining causing internal blisters and ulcers. Some oils can also cause organ damage when taken internally, this has even resulted in death. Put simply ingesting oils is not worth the risk!

With regards to the 'organic' label; essential oils fall under cosmetics rather than food or pharmaceuticals. Therefore the terms 'pure' and 'organic' mean nothing, there is no legislation protecting these terms when used in cosmetics, meaning any cosmetic can claim to be 'organic'. These terms are simply a marketing term, if you really want to check a cosmetic/essential oil is organic then seek out ones which carry the Soil Association logo. Whilst essential oils made from organically grown plants may have environmental benefits, the jury is still out as to whether the oil itself has a better therapeutic value and therefore standard safety advice still applies.

Some essential oils are not suitable for people with certain medical conditions, including pregnancy or when taking medications so please check each oil you intend to use. Also extra caution needs to be taken when using oils with children, several should be avoided and dilutions are higher. Guidelines constantly change around this issue and since this guide in intended for adults, seek the latest advise if you wish to use oils on children.

Some oils are also more prone to cause sensitisation in people e.g. cause rashes due to overuse. This is why it is advised to use oils sparingly (remember less is more!) and to not keep using the same oils repeatedly.

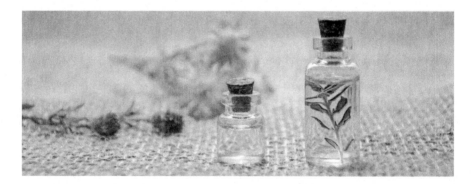

Essential Oil Usage

Probably the most common way to use essential oils at home is using a diffuser; either one with a tea light or an electric steam diffuser. Personally I prefer a steam diffuser as they do not use heat which can degrade the oil, meaning the oil smells stronger. Always follow manufacturers instructions but for either diffusers usually 5-6 drops of oil added to water is all that is needed to ll your room with fragrance.

If you wish to use oils on your skin, remember they need to be diluted, usually to around 2% value (i.e. 2ml of total essential oil in 98ml of base product) Aromatherapy suppliers have a whole range of base products you can add oils to including carrier oils, creams, shampoos and shower gels.

If using in a bath, please remember water and oil do not mix! Your oils still need diluting in a base bath product and then adding to the water. Without such, the essential oil will float on the surface of the water and come into contact with your skin on getting in the bath. I see many well-meaning recipes online advising people to mix oils with bath salts, however they do not mix very well either. By all means throw in a handful of epsom/Himalayan salts into your bath but add your essential oils in a suitable base separately.

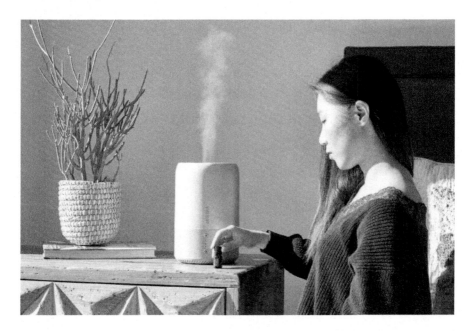

Thank You!

I hope you have found this book informative and have gained ideas on how you can improve your sleep.

I'd love to hear your feedback and do let me know if there are any other titles you would like to see in the series via social media.

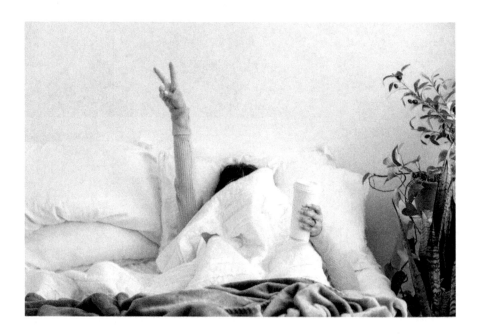

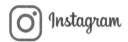 Instagram

@leruwellness

Printed in Great Britain
by Amazon

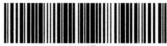

22488614R00046